Autophagy:

10 Powerful Secrets of Healing and Anti-Aging Through a Power of Waterfasting. Learn How You Can Burn Fat Very Easily!

© Copyright 2019 by Chantel Stephens - All rights reserved.

This content is provided with the sole purpose of providing relevant information on a specific topic for which every reasonable effort has been made to ensure that it is both accurate and reasonable. Nevertheless, by purchasing this content you consent to the fact that the author, as well as the publisher, are in no way experts on the topics contained herein, regardless of any claims as such that may be made within. As such, any suggestions or recommendations that are made within are done so purely for entertainment value. It is recommended that you always consult a professional prior to undertaking any of the advice or techniques discussed within.

This is a legally binding declaration that is considered both valid and fair by both the Committee of Publishers Association and the American Bar Association and should be considered as legally binding within the United States.

The reproduction, transmission, and duplication of any of the content found herein, including any specific or extended information will be done as an illegal act regardless of the end form the information ultimately takes. This includes copied versions of the work both physical, digital and audio unless express consent of the Publisher is provided beforehand. Any additional rights reserved.

Furthermore, the information that can be found within the pages described forthwith shall be considered both accurate and truthful when it comes to the recounting of facts. As such, any use, correct or incorrect, of the provided information will render the Publisher free of responsibility as to the actions taken outside of their direct purview. Regardless, there are zero scenarios where the original author or the Publisher can be deemed liable in any fashion for any damages or hardships that may result from any of the information discussed herein.

Additionally, the information in the following pages is intended only for informational purposes and should thus be thought of as universal. As befitting its nature, it is presented without assurance regarding its prolonged validity or interim quality. Trademarks that are mentioned are done without written consent and can in no way be considered an endorsement from the trademark holder.

Table of Contents

Introduction......5
Chapter 1: What is Autophagy?......8
Chapter 2: The science of autophagy made simple......16
Chapter 3: To fast, or not to fast—potential benefits, drawbacks and risks......28
Chapter 4: Fasting—how to begin, and what to expect......44
Chapter 5: Autophagy for your lifestyle......52
Chapter 6: Autophagy and weight loss......81
Chapter 7: Autophagy and the aging process......88
Chapter 8: Autophagy and health disorders......95
Chapter 9: Autophagy and the mind......100
Conclusion......102

Introduction

Congratulations on purchasing this copy of *Autophagy: 10 Powerful Secrets of Healing and Anti-Aging Through a Power of Waterfasting. Learn How You Can Burn Fast Very Easily!*
, and thank you for doing so. Within the following chapters, you'll find explanations of the process known as "autophagy," in-depth analysis of its benefits, drawbacks, and risks, as well as the guidance needed to begin incorporating autophagy into your lifestyle, if you should decide that it's the right choice for your body.

Autophagy is a term commonly associated with fasting for the sake of health and wellness, though it's important to note that the word is not synonymous with fasting. Autophagy refers to a particular cellular pathway that exists within our bodies, a process which may be triggered or bolstered by restricted caloric intake—but this process can also take place automatically, within a body that maintains a regular diet of three meals (or more) each day. Autophagy is the natural mechanism of waste disposal and toxin removal that the cells in our bodies use to keep things running smoothly; it happens inside of all of us, whether we are fitness buffs or couch potatoes; whether we are militant macrobiotic vegans, or red-meat and dark liquor enthusiasts; whether we are young or old, male or female or non-binary, we all have used this process to maintain our health at the cellular level, without ever being aware of it.

The real crux of the issue is that autophagy doesn't always work as efficiently as we'd like it to when left to its own devices; often, it becomes less effective over time, as we age, or as a reflection of certain lifestyle habits. When it grows lazy, slow-acting, or ineffectual, autophagy eventually needs a boost, coming in the form of caloric restriction or manufactured cellular stress, such as extreme physical exertion. Recent studies have found that regular induction of autophagy can do a great deal more than simply help people to lose weight or feel better about their physical appearance—in fact, it may be linked to improved organ function, reduced inflammation and pain, metabolic regulation, disease prevention, cancer cures, and increased longevity.

This is why interest in the process, and how we can induce and best control it through purposeful behaviors, has grown so much in recent decades. Autophagy is like an internal fountain of youth locked inside every one of us—only we haven't quite managed to find the right key to unlock its secrets yet. Most research done thus far on autophagy has been performed on animals, not humans, so there is still a great deal that the scientific and medical communities are not yet certain of. This being the case, it's important to recognize that autophagy may not be safe or ideal for everyone; even after reading this book, you should consult a medical professional before embarking on any type of extreme fast (exceeding 24 hours, or exceeding 16 hours if done on a regular basis) to ensure the process of inducing autophagy will be helpful and healing rather than harmful. This book was written for informational purposes and should not be taken as medical advice; rather, any concepts within this book that seem particularly relevant to your experience should be brought up and explored in your next appointment with your doctor.

There are plenty of books on this subject on the market, so thank you again for choosing this one! Every effort was made to ensure it is full of as much useful and accurate information as possible; please enjoy!

Chapter 1: What is Autophagy?

The term "autophagy" was first coined in 1963 by Belgian biochemist Christian de Duve while studying insulin. It was an accidental discovery, not the primary focus of his work, but having been the first to identify this cellular pathway, he was able to assign a name to it. The term derives from two Greek words: "auto," meaning "self," and "phagein," meaning "to eat." Yes, you read that correctly: autophagy means self-eating or self-consuming.

But rest assured—there is nothing inherently gross or cannibalistic about this concept. Autophagy occurs at the cellular level—mostly inside your body, but it also works on your skin, which is an organ just like your liver or heart. Christian de Duve's discovery was that this process occurs within all living organisms as a sort of self-cleansing maintenance system, working to eliminate damaged cell matter so that the remaining matter can function at a heightened level of efficiency. While some cells within the body use apoptosis, a process of organized self-destruction, to combat internal damage or malfunction, autophagy is a cellular pathway that allows cells to repair their own internal damage, replace broken parts as needed, and thrive in spite of challenges, promoting cellular adaptability. It happens automatically, whether we aim to activate the process or not, though its degree of effectiveness may fluctuate throughout our lifetimes and be impacted by diet, environmental factors, stress levels, and more.

Without this process, no individual cell can survive for long, just as we humans couldn't survive without our own system of waste elimination and toxin filtration. When autophagy begins to slow or fail to work on a grand scale, it can lead to cellular death, which may ultimately result in the death of the host organism. By contrast, when autophagy is bolstered by certain lifestyle habits and activities, it can have a rejuvenating effect, extending the lifespan of cells and, theoretically, the bodies that these cells comprise.

It wasn't until 1983, twenty years after the initial discovery, that Yoshinori Ohsumi was able to discover the specific genes that control autophagy. Ohsumi performed a series of research experiments on baker's yeast, aiming to gain further insight into the mechanism of autophagy within the microorganism—but his work proved to be revolutionary to the biological, medical, health and wellness industries over the next few decades, and ended up earning him a Nobel Prize in 2016, because he was able to draw a comparison between the function of autophagy in yeast cells and the cells of the human body. His discoveries opened doorways in the world of cancer research, infectious disease, and neurodegenerative disorders; they provided insight into many previously mysterious physiological processes, such as the way our bodies work in starvation mode, or our cellular responses to environmental stressors.

Autophagy doesn't only work to remove toxic buildup and waste from the cell; it also uses this material as an alternative source of fuel for energy. In that way, it is very much like a cellular recycling system, making the most of every damaged protein and broken down organelle, pushing the body to become more energy efficient. It also serves to make cells more resilient, improving immune function and boosting both disease and infection resistance. Autophagy helps to promote and maintain homeostasis, which is the body's ability to maintain stability and equilibrium at the cellular level.

While it's still challenging to monitor levels of autophagic activity in human bodies, one thing we do know for certain is that autophagy happens automatically, and works most efficiently, when we are young, without being triggered by any unusual dietary habits or extreme levels of physical exertion. At this point, autophagy works at a moderate level, in "maintenance mode," essentially doing only as much cellular cleanup as is necessary. It is only over time, as we collect more and more cellular damage in our bodies to gunk up the works, that the process of autophagy can begin to lag and grow ineffective at preventing or repairing damage. After this point, the best way to reactivate autophagy is by introducing cellular stress; this is because autophagy only increases when it is in "stress-response mode" rather than "maintenance mode," and for that to happen, the cells must detect a veritable threat, such as nutrition scarcity.

It's possible that autophagy functions differently in humans as compared to other animals, which is why further research is necessary before we can make any claims or offer any instruction with absolute certainty as to their accuracy. Most conclusive research on this process has thus far been performed on non-human species, such as mice, insects, and microscopic organisms. Still, some of its beneficial effects, such as weight loss, improved complexion, or reduced inflammation, can be witnessed and experienced in real time, as purposefully activated autophagy can produce these results fairly quickly.

Why does autophagy exist?

The evolution of autophagy as it relates to human biological history and anthropology has not yet been extensively studied, but based on its apparent preventative correlation to modern age diseases, we can draw some interesting theories as to its initial evolutionary purpose. Autophagy seems to work strongest in a body that is in danger of starvation, or responding to other potentially mortal threats. Most of the activities and factors that bolster it happen to align closely with those habits that our pre-agricultural ancestors would have enacted through a hunter-gatherer lifestyle. We can theorize, then, that human autophagy was an evolutionary development designed to ensure survival in the face of nutritional scarcity, predatory threats, and a general lack of stability or predictability.

This ties neatly into the theories that have inspired the paleo diet and lifestyle trend, which is similar to the ketogenic diet in practice. Paleo is built upon the notion that our bodies have not evolved or changed much, physiologically speaking, since the era in which they were designed by evolution to make the most of a paleolithic landscape. Our ancestors would not have needed to efficiently digest processed foods or farmed grains; therefore, it is logical to conclude that our modern bodies are stressed, inflamed, obese and sick because they aren't designed to handle the diets, activities, and environmental factors we currently expose them to. Likewise, we can deduce that since our hunter-gatherer ancestors would often live for days at a time without much (or any) food, only to feast to their satisfaction upon the completion of a successful hunt, it isn't likely that our bodies are designed to function on a steady, constant stream of caloric intake, nor that they are designed to be intolerant of an occasional binge after a fasting period.

It's entirely possible that within the human body, autophagy exists not only as a restorative process, but as a survival mechanism as well. When the body goes into starvation mode, autophagy works quickly to remove any cellular waste that could become a tax on the body if health begins to fail; it also works to enhance energy levels and promote alertness, ambitious drive, mental clarity, and even sensory perceptions, such as heightened sensitivity to sound, all to ensure that the body is in prime condition for a successful hunt. In the present day, those of us who are lucky enough to have steady incomes almost never find ourselves worrying about where our next meal will come from. The skills that we once developed for the paleolithic world have been rendered unnecessary and incompatible with the modern landscape. Our internal clocks and circadian rhythms have fallen out of sync with our scheduling demands; our digestive systems are ill-equipped to handle the refined carbohydrates and sugar that we consistently consume. Most of us lead lives wherein comfort and satiety have become the norm rather than the exception to the rule, and generally speaking, our autophagic responses have grown lethargic and ineffective through lack of use.

Of course, we all want to feel safe, satisfied, and secure—any threat that poses a challenge to our continued survival or comfort is easily vilified. But suppose the human body has evolved specifically to handle the uncertainty of a world without grocery stores, or reliable schedules, or even doors with locks on them? Suppose the body evolved to manage a form of physical stress that modern life no longer provides for us? Is it possible that, by making food sources ubiquitous and easily accessible, we mistakenly shortchanged our own bodies, exchanging our physical health for the possibility of achieving peace of mind?

There is indeed evidence to suggest that even in the early days of the agricultural revolution, the incorporation of farmed grain into the human diet took a great toll on the height and overall health levels of the population. Studies of these ancient skeletons show that early agriculturalists struggled to adapt to the stress of their new lifestyle, encountering new infectious diseases and severe nutritional deficiencies. And contrary to popular belief, their nomadic predecessors were not uniformly condemned to early, gruesome deaths; many hunter-gatherers of the paleolithic era were able to survive well into their seventies without encountering chronic diseases or fatal cancers.

These facts inform the theory behind using induced autophagy as a treatment for those chronic diseases and disorders that seem to be increasing in frequency and severity in correlation to the progression of modern agriculture. The disorders that pose the greatest threats to modern Americans, causing the highest rates of preventable mortality, are (in order of prevalence): heart disease; cancer; chronic lower respiratory disease (often as a result of smoking tobacco); accidental injury; stroke; Alzheimer's disease; and diabetes. Excluding accidental injuries, all of these killers are facts of modern life; there is almost no evidence that these illnesses and conditions were prevalent amongst our hunter-gatherer ancestors. Furthermore, we can lessen our chances of falling victim to any and all of these killers (including accidental injury, this time) by maintaining healthy levels of autophagic activity throughout our lives.

Chapter 2: The science of autophagy made simple

In order to truly understand the process of autophagy, one must build upon some basic knowledge of the way that the human body works at the physiological and cellular levels. You do not need to be an expert in biology, anatomy, or any other branch of science to comprehend these concepts, but the scientific terminology used in this book may be difficult to make sense of without previous study in cellular biology or other related sciences.

In this chapter, we'll outline some of the terms and concepts of cellular biology and metabolic functions, with specialized focus on those terms which are most relevant to our discussion of autophagy. We'll explain them in layman's terms, assuming that you have no prior background in biology or previous understanding of the cellular life cycle.

A lexicon for autophagy

Cells

This term is probably familiar to you, but we'll review it just to ensure that the rest of the terminology in this chapter makes sense. Cells are the building blocks of life. They are the smallest functional unit within any living organism. There are smaller units, but they do not function on their own as cells do; you might think of the cell as a vehicle, which can be disassembled into smaller metal parts—but none of these metal parts can travel on its own. Cells can be eukaryotic or prokaryotic—typically, eukaryotic cells are parts of larger microorganisms and contain several membrane bound organelles, while prokaryotic cells are often single-cell organisms without any distinct internal organelles. An example of a eukaryotic cell is a cell found within a flower, a tree, a spider, a rhinoceros, a mushroom, or a human being; meanwhile, prokaryotic cells are found in bacteria or archaea.

Nucleus

Each eukaryotic cell contains a nucleus, which is often thought of as the brain of a cell. It is responsible for storing the cell's genetic information, and for managing all activity throughout the rest of the cell body.

Cytoplasm

The cytoplasm is a gelatinous substance that fills the rest of the cell outside of the nucleus. Organelles are contained within the cytoplasm.

Organelles

These are the parts of the cell which may be disassembled and repurposed in the process of autophagy. You might think of them as the organs of a cell; there are a variety of types which all serve different functions and purposes.

Mitochondria

This organelle is responsible for cellular respiration, and is often referred to as the power house or power plant of the cell. Autophagy is believed to help cells to build stronger, more efficient mitochondria, leading to overall higher energy levels. Rates of mitochondrial turnover are closely related to aging and longevity.

Vacuoles

These are membrane-bound organelles that play a crucial role in the process of autophagy, promoting a balance between regeneration and degradation of cellular matter, preventing bottlenecks caused by overproduction and inefficient waste disposal, and aiding in the process of recycling misfolded proteins.

Lysosomes

This particular organelle contains enzymes that serve a special purpose: they can break down damaged proteins. Some refer to the lysosome as the stomach of a cell, but for the purposes of autophagic study, it might help to think of it instead as the cell's garbage disposal and recycling center, all in one. During autophagy, suboptimal cell matter is packaged into little membrane sacks, like garbage bags, which are then dropped off with the lysosome to degrade their contents and dispose of them.

Autophagosomes

This is the word for the specific membrane sack, or garbage bag, that is used in autophagy to sequester damaged cell matter (such as an old, broken down organelle, or a damaged protein) and then transport it to the lysosome for degradation.

Vesicles

A vesicle is a type of vacuole that is filled with fluid and encased by a lipid bilayer. Vesicles work to transport fluids from one cell to another, or simply to store substances until a later time, at which point they might be useful to the cell. The autophagic process makes use of vesicles to transport material to the lysosome, but vesicles are also used in other cellular pathways for differing purposes.

Cell division

This is the process through which cells reproduce, dividing themselves into two or more daughter cells, each containing genetic information from the parent cell. The daughter cells can either be genetically identical to the parent, or receive only half of the parent cell's genetic information. This reproductive process is how organisms work to replace dead, senescent, or malfunctioning cells to extend the lifespan of the host organism.

During cell division, a major concern is the parent cell's ability to maintain genomic integrity; genetic mutations from cell division can cause a number of problems, including unchecked cell growth without homeostatic limitation, or, by contrast, promoting apoptosis. Cancerous cells also grow and reproduce through this same process; so, when we aim to use autophagy to promote healthy cellular development, we also run the risk of encouraging reproduction of corrupted, malfunctioning, and dangerous cells.

When cells are no longer able to divide and reproduce, they become senescent, which essentially means that they are not quite dead yet, but they aren't functioning or working to serve the intracellular system. When a cell becomes senescent, it sends out signals to other cells in the body, basically requesting to be destroyed through apoptosis or autophagy. This is often a good thing, as it can prevent damaged cells and genetic mutations from replicating and spreading throughout the body, causing disease.

Free radicals

In the world of chemistry, a radical is defined as any molecule, atom or ion that has an unpaired valence electron; the lack of pairing makes them highly reactive and volatile, as they prefer to be in a paired state. You might think of a free radical as a highly codependent person who has just been dumped by their romantic partner before attending a dinner party at which they are the only uncoupled attendee. Under normal circumstances, they might be a perfectly lovely person to spend time with, but in a free radical state, having just lost the partner upon which they are dependent, their behavior may become unpredictable, desperate, volatile, and damaging to those around them.

Free radicals in the body will aggressively search for a new electron to pair with. They are scavengers, and don't see any problem with stealing those desired electrons from otherwise healthy and high-functioning cells or proteins. When they do so, they may cause cell mutation and interrupt cellular homeostasis.

Free radicals can be produced by normal metabolic processes within the body, but they can also be introduced by external factors, such as a diet full of processed foods and preservatives, excessive alcohol consumption, or exposure to environmental hazards like cigarette smoke, harsh UV rays, pesticides, and air pollutants. You cannot ever extract all free radicals from your body, nor can you prevent free radical damage entirely—in fact, to a small degree, it is a necessary ingredient in a well-functioning organism—but *excessive* buildup of free radicals in the body can be dangerous to your overall health.

Oxidative stress

The damage that free radicals cause to the body is often referred to as "oxidative stress" or "oxidative damage." When oxygen molecules split within the body through the process of oxygen metabolism (which is normal and not preventable), they initiate oxidation, during which they will aim to steal electrons from any available source.

When we expose our bodies to large amounts of free radicals, the chance that they will damage or corrupt healthy proteins, DNA and molecules within the body is heightened. This is why many adults consume antioxidant-rich foods in hopes of combatting this process and lowering their chances of causing chronic disease or cancer through oxidative stress. The body has natural defenses to use against free radical damage, and these defenses can be bolstered by certain positive dietary and lifestyle choices (eating colorful fruits and vegetables, for instance, or supplements like vitamin E and selenium), but our bodies can usually only handle a certain workload before these defense systems are rendered ineffective. Our natural defenses against oxidative stress are weakened over time as we age. This can be a vicious cycle, as free radical buildup can inhibit signals that promote autophagy, which would otherwise work to combat oxidative stress.

Lipolysis

Lipolysis is the metabolic process through which fats and other lipids are broken down and converted into glycerol and fatty acids, after which point they can be released into the bloodstream. If a body has an excess of stored fat, lipolysis works to mobilize it and use it for energy. High insulin levels can interfere with the process of lipolysis, whereas low insulin levels trigger both autophagy and lipolysis to work cooperatively. Lipolysis is the primary goal of following a ketogenic diet, while ketosis (the creation of ketones as a byproduct of lipolysis) is it's secondary objective.

Insulin

Insulin is a hormone that allows the body to either use glucose (simple sugars that the body extracts from carbohydrates that we eat) for energy, or store it within organs and cells for future use. It extracts glucose from the bloodstream; this is the "blood sugar" we often refer to in relation to insulin resistance and conditions like diabetes. It is produced in the pancreas as a response to heightened levels of glucose in the blood after we eat; if we overeat for extended periods of time, the body may become desensitized to its release, or "insulin resistant," which can wreak havoc on almost every system in the body, as the pancreas continues producing insulin to very little effect. A spike in insulin is typically caused by an overabundance or buildup of glucose in the bloodstream. Prolonged periods of high insulin levels may promote development of many different kinds of malignancies in the body, whereas a drop in insulin levels triggers increased autophagy and improved metabolic health.

Anabolism and catabolism

Whenever you read up on strategies for muscle growth, weight loss, or muscular stamina on the cellular level, you're likely to hear the words "anabolic" and "catabolic" frequently. Anabolism references processes that build up new matter within the body, whereas catabolism references processes that degrade and break down matter for digestion, recycling, or disposal. Autophagy is a catabolic process, while digesting food to extract energy from it is an anabolic process.

Apoptosis

This is the process of cellular death within an intracellular program; unlike in necrosis, where cells die from injury, apoptosis is sometimes referred to as "cellular suicide" because it happens in an orderly and efficient manner. Components of the cell are broken down into smaller pieces and eliminated as waste. In this process, the cell self-destructs as an automatic response to certain triggers, often to the benefit of other related cells. Apoptosis destroys the entirety of the cell, whereas in autophagy, damaged parts of the cell may be replaced one at a time, as needed. Both apoptosis and autophagy are popular concepts in the realm of medical science and disease prevention, and for similar reasons; either controlled cell death, or triggered cell restoration and regeneration, could be revolutionary to cancer treatment, for example, so long as we are able to predict, manufacture, monitor and govern these processes in human patients with accuracy and consistency.

mTOR

Mammalian Target of Rapamycin, or mTOR, is a pathway that stimulates cellular growth and anabolic processes, and regulates nutrient signaling within the body. Whenever it senses an overabundance of energy (usually after eating), it will work to send that energy to the places where it is needed most. When the body is well-fed, it works to prohibit autophagy by binding with a kinase that can trigger the process; when the body is low on nutrients, mTOR releases its grip on this kinase, freeing it up to activate autophagy again. Hyperactivity of mTOR may be related to development of neurodegenerative disease or tumor growth; by contrast, suppression of mTOR has been proven effective at extending the lifespans of some rodents, bacteria, and a few different yeast species. Tools and strategies to inhibit mTOR are quite similar to those one might use to induce autophagy. Over-suppression of mTOR should be avoided, though, as it can lead to muscular degeneration and atrophy.

Telomeres

A telomere is the structure that protects the ends of your chromosomes and prevents them from sticking together during cell division. They are relevant to autophagy and anti-aging because they protect genetic information during cell division and allow the process to continue. Each time a cell divides, a small piece of the chromosome is lost, ultimately shortening its length; when the chromosome becomes too short, the cell can no longer divide, and thus becomes inactive or senescent, ultimately leading to cell death. Longer telomeres may not prevent this type of cellular death, but they can help to prolong the division process, and stave off external signs of aging and cancer development at the cellular level. On the other hand, when telomeres are too long, they can actually serve to help cancer cells survive through aggressive treatments like chemotherapy, essentially making them invincible. You can keep your telomeres long through stress management, regular exercise, maintenance of a healthy diet, and adequate restorative sleep.

How does autophagy work?

Once you understand some of the more intimidating scientific terms involved, the process of autophagy can be understood quite easily. When activated by stressors, such as nutrient deprivation, autophagy first works to identify any organic material in the body (proteins, organelles, etc) that has become, or could potentially become, an energetic drain to the cellular system. It then works to sequester the threatening material within vesicles (or autophagosomes, more specifically) and then transport it therein to the lysosome, where it can then assist in the degradation of these particles. Finally, it works to restructure or repurpose these broken down particles to generate energy, or recycle the materials for use in cell repair. It is a system of automated resourcefulness, helping to improve the body's current genetic material rather than killing and replacing inefficient parts.

Imagine your body as a house built in summertime (let the season represent your youth); in warm and sunny conditions, you might open all the windows and doors, allowing wind to sweep freely through the building. But as winter approaches and the winds grow colder, you'll be faced with a choice: either find a way to secure the house's barriers and trap heat inside or ditch the house and head someplace warmer to start rebuilding. Autophagy is like the voice in your head that motivates you to close and seal all the windows, and perhaps even chop up the wood from that broken closet door and burn it in the fireplace, saving you a great deal of money and energy, and sparing you from the inconvenience and risk of having to start all over.

There are different categorical types of autophagy; because it is a multi-step process, it can be used within the body to serve different functions, and can be triggered and influenced by a wide variety of external stimulus factors. Many of these factors and their potential impact on the autophagic process are not yet fully understood, which is why further scientific study of autophagy is required before it can be used in routine medical treatment. What we do know for sure, though, is that controlled nutrient deprivation works to promote autophagy, and a lack of cellular stress works to inhibit it, weakening and suppressing the process more and more as we age.

Chapter 3: To fast, or not to fast—potential benefits, drawbacks and risks

Both intermittent and extreme fasting have become quite popular within the health and wellness community over the last decade, along with dietary and lifestyle trends like the Paleo diet, Ketogenic Diet, and Epigenetic diet. Some have even built entire brand empires devoted to promoting autophagy as the secret ingredient to a long, satisfying and successful life.

But with so many people singing its praises and declaring it to be a panacea, it is important to be aware that autophagy is something of double-edged blade; while studies have hinted at its incredible restorative and healing abilities, there are also some case studies that expose the dangers of overactive autophagy. In short, too much of it can actually make you sicker, rather than healing you. This being the case, it is imperative that you do your research before embarking on any extreme fasting or exercise regimen, and when you do experiment, be sure to remain attentive to your body's signals.

Potential benefits of autophagy induction

Weight loss

Many health and wellness experts are adamant that the primary benefit of autophagy is its restorative and rejuvenating capabilities—but undoubtedly, weight loss is a highly desirable side effect that can be achieved through regular induction of the process. Many people who have struggled with weight management over the course of decades, and who have tried virtually every dietary trend under the sun, report that it is both easier to drop excess fat and easier to keep it off by promoting autophagy, rather than by simply following a restricted calorie diet and increasing aerobic exercise. Contrary to popular belief, it is far easier to maintain a healthy bodyweight through regular autophagic activation than through extreme dieting, primarily because intermittent fasting and macronutrient management do not impair metabolic function over time, nor do they require you to constantly avoid caloric satiety. Traditional weight loss plans often rely on the individual's ability to consistently reduce caloric intake in order to avoid plateaus or repeated weight gain, but this is unsustainable and requires an unrealistic degree of self-discipline. Many people prefer to fast and look forward to an eventual feast, rather than living in a perpetual state of hunger and craving suppression.

There are also those who believe autophagic induction to be preferable to traditional diet and exercise as a means of losing large amounts of weight, because autophagy seems to simultaneously utilize stored fat and unneeded cells in the skin for energy, erasing the need for body lift surgeries or other extreme and costly treatments for removal of sagging, excess skin; instead, the skin appears to manage its own shrinkage gradually, and does so at a rate that is compatible to the speed of weight loss, restoring and maintaining its elasticity.

Glowing, youthful complexion

Even if excess skin post-weight loss isn't a concern for you, induced autophagy can still provide numerous benefits to the skin. For the young, it can combat inflammation, as well as eliminate bacteria and other toxins that cause blemishes, cysts, boils, skin infections, and even conditions like eczema and psoriasis. For the elderly, it can also work to rejuvenate skin cells, keeping them elastic and resilient, preventing wrinkles, dullness and discoloration. Whatever your age, autophagy appears to promote a smoother, softer, more radiant complexion.

Reliable energy

Autophagy doesn't only promote higher energy levels; it also serves to regulate and maintain energy levels in a long-term sense, by improving the function of mitochondria and training cells to source energy from damaged material already found within, rather than having to extract glucose from the bloodstream. If you've ever done a fad diet, chances are you are familiar with the intense energy crashes and mood swings that come from relying exclusively on carbohydrate consumption for temporary doses of energy. Altering your lifestyle to consistently bolster the process of autophagy will effectively break the cycle of addiction to glucose energy and retrain your body to function at high levels in the absence of caloric intake. It can also teach the body to use the act of feasting to promote rest in the evening, rather than to fuel a few hours' worth of stamina three times each day.

Curbed sugar cravings

When autophagy is at its best, cells are less desperate to pull sugar from the bloodstream to source their own energy; instead, they look within themselves and become resourceful, destroying their own damaged parts and repurposing them. Over time, and with consistency, this will train the body to break its addiction to sweets and dampen the intensity of sugar cravings.

Less body odor

Autophagy primes the body to eliminate toxins quickly and efficiently. Our bodies have other methods for toxin extraction and removal, such as sweating or urinating them out. Those who induce autophagy regularly find that they have lower internal toxin levels overall, and thus their sweat, urine, saliva, and other bodily fluids contain a great deal less of the bacteria that typically cause these fluids to carry foul odors.

Improved muscle performance

The more often our bodies practice autophagy, the better they get at it, eventually training most cells within the body to become more energy efficient and resilient. These qualities make it much easier to build and use muscle tissue; by contrast, low levels of autophagy can contribute to degeneration of muscle fibers.

Reduced inflammation

Much of the time, inflammation is caused by a buildup of old, broken down cellular junk left in the body. Autophagy makes use of this junk, burning it for energy and helping to remove it from the body, reducing issues like swelling of organs or joints, aches and pains, severe itches and rashes, and other forms of inflammation stemming from autoimmune dysfunction or infection.

No more bloating

Many of us have come to accept frequent bloating as an unavoidable fact of life, but in truth, bloating is usually a sign that some part of the digestive tract isn't working as smoothly or efficiently as it's supposed to. It's often an indication of inflammation from food allergies or intolerance, infections or chronic diseases impacting the digestive system. Autophagy works to reduce that inflammation and heal damage to the digestive organs. Furthermore, it promotes the dissolution of fat into fatty acids, which are flushed from the body in the form of water, preventing bloating from excess water retention. Finally, it promotes overall gut health, which can help to ensure regularity of bowel movements and prevent constipation, so long as the body is adequately hydrated.

Regulated metabolic function

Intermittent and extreme fasting to trigger autophagy can also do a great deal to reverse conditions like insulin resistance, hypoglycemia, prediabetes, or type 2 diabetes by teaching cells to reduce their dependence on sugar for energy.

Boosted immune system

The immune system is complex, and requires a lot of energy in order to do its job well. Autophagy helps all waste and toxin eliminating organs to function better, allowing more energy to be diverted to the immune system's pursuit of infectious organisms and other potential threats to your health. Furthermore, when your cells are well-practiced at consuming the weakest parts of themselves, they become extremely efficient and can quickly and easily use the same strategy to fight off invaders, like infection.

Faster healing

Autophagy makes your cells more resilient, and better able to withstand stress and recover from injury or illness. When induced regularly, it should allow you to bounce back from most any setback fairly quickly, at least in comparison to the average recovery time. By inducing autophagy, we can trick our bodies into believing that there is some form of imminent threat to our survival, and the body responds, mercifully, by doing everything in its power to set us up for successful hunting or escape from a predator. This doesn't mean that autophagy can cure a broken bone overnight, but it does mean that it will streamline all biological processes in the body to promote the fastest possible recovery from any injury, infection, or disease.

Enhanced cognitive function

Though initial attempts at fasting to induce autophagy may induce brain fog, as the body goes into carbohydrate withdrawal, in the long run, autophagy is found to promote mental clarity and higher levels of cognitive function.

The connection between the gut and the mind is profound. Both organs are connected by the vagus nerve, so dysfunction on either end can have a negative cyclical effect on the body, with an inflamed gut causing decreased brain function and decreased brain function leading to poor or impulsive dietary and lifestyle choices, which then further disrupt the function of digestive organs in turn. Autophagy not only works to reduce reliance on carbohydrate energy and inflammation in the digestive tract; it also allows each organ in your body to function more efficiently and independently, essentially removing sources of biological distraction from the brain's workload.

Additionally, autophagy works to counteract the buildup of damaged molecules, misfolded proteins, and senescent cells that are believed to spur the development of neurodegenerative diseases, dementia, and loss of neuroplasticity in old age. Finally, when the body is in a state of nutritional starvation and charged by adequate restorative rest, autophagy can boost our alertness, sensory perceptions, reaction times, and mental acuity; it can even serve to improve memory. All this is done to ensure the body will be able to locate and secure food in the face of nutritional scarcity, and to escape predators. If hunting, or running away from a hungry predator, isn't a priority for you, the cognitive benefits of autophagy activation can still be easily applied to other challenges that are more relevant to modern life.

Better quality sleep

Many of us believe that the length of time we spend sleeping each night is what matters most, but when it comes to improving health outcomes, what truly counts is how much *restorative sleep* we get. This type of rest, also called deep sleep or REM sleep, is the type that promotes restoration, healing, and rejuvenation at the cellular level. For most adults, it's only about a quarter of the time we spend in bed, and it may be less than that if poor health conditions cause interruptions to your sleep cycle. Autophagy can improve sleep quality by reversing these health conditions. It also helps to regulate metabolic function, which influences our circadian rhythms by effecting body temperature, appetite and energy levels. Autophagy may not necessarily prompt you to sleep longer, but it may allow you to sleep for fewer hours and awake feeling even more restored and energized.

Fight psychiatric disorders

It appears that autophagy may be able to play a role in treatment of disorders such as clinical depression, bipolar disorder, or even schizophrenia. This theory still needs to be put to further experimentation, but the evidence in favor of it is compelling. In tests on rats, autophagy was found to have a distinct anti-depressant effect. Furthermore, post-mortem analyses of patient's brains have shown a clear link between interrupted or failed autophagy and schizophrenia, as well as a number of related neurodegenerative diseases, implying a potential causal link.

Combat neurodegenerative illness and dementia

Autophagy stimulates growth of new cellular matter, particularly matter that is needed to build nerve and brain cells, enhancing neuroplasticity;

in essence, it works to keep our brain cells young and healthy. While there is some concern that autophagy is not yet well enough understood and controlled for use in cancer treatment, as in some cases the cancerous cells may hijack the process and use it to their own advantage, it seems to be much less risky to use autophagy induction to combat diseases like Alzheimer's and Parkinson's. These neurodegenerative conditions are caused by a buildup of damaged protein in and around neurons, interrupting neural pathways; but autophagy can effectively degrade and eliminate this protein buildup, much like an electric toothbrush dislodging and removing plaque buildup from the gums and teeth; and in this case, there is no risk of the damaged proteins hijacking the autophagic process for the sake of their own survival, as a cancerous cell might.

Disease prevention

It's believed that autophagy can be most powerful as a preventative practice, helping to stop developing diseases and chronic disorders in their tracks before they have the chance to grow severe. It detoxifies cells and repairs damage from environmental stressors and free radicals that may cause health complications. Autophagy can help to lower cholesterol levels and blood pressure, conditions which can contribute to failing health. It also works to combat oxidative stress, inflammation, and infection, all of which can lead to the development of chronic pain and disease.

Cancer prevention and treatment

Research in this area is still ongoing, and results are as of yet inconclusive. It seems very promising that autophagy may be a key factor in prevention and lowering rates of recurrence for those in remission; studies on human breast cancer patients have shown a dramatic reduction of recurrence rates amongst those who regularly practiced autophagy over a period of roughly ten years. Many are hopeful that we can harness this same restorative and regenerative power to fight active cancer cells and combat cancer growth, but until we are better able to measure and control autophagy, it will remain risky for cancer patients to use fasting as an element of their treatment regimens. Active cancer cells are sometimes able to use autophagy to their own advantage, growing stronger and more resistant to treatments.

Longevity

One particularly bright, shining beacon of hope in the study of autophagy is the "impossible" promise it holds: restored youth and extended lifespan. Studies show that the inhibition of autophagy is closely linked to cell degeneration, which is what prompts signs of aging and generalized health decline, so it stands to reason that by strengthening autophagy, we might be able to pause, prevent, or even reverse this process.

Potential drawbacks

Insufficient research

The discovery of autophagy and the genetic components that govern it are quite recent, relatively speaking. Very little research has been performed involving human subjects, and in order to observe the long-term effects of autophagy on health and longevity, we would need to have discovered it more than five or six decades ago. Despite Yoshinori Ohsumi's extensive work, autophagy still exists as something of a black box mystery; while we can observe what we believe to be resulting effects of it, we are still unable to effectively measure the process within the human body, limiting our understanding of potential strategic applications.

No testing methods

Currently, no methods exist to be able to test autophagy levels in living humans. We can measure some adjacent signifiers, such as ketone or glucose levels in the bloodstream or urine, but there is no test available at this point which can conclusively tell you how efficiently autophagy is (or is not) working in your body. This makes it very difficult even for experts to say decisively which lifestyle changes can have the greatest impact on autophagic activity, or to know precisely how much fasting, exercise, or cellular stress is ideal for different body types, age groups, genders, or other demographic groups.

Can be easily overdone

One major difficulty we face, having no effective way to measure autophagy within the human body, is that we can't always predict when this process is working effectively and being helpful, or when it is in hyperdrive, perhaps doing more harm than good. When extreme fasting or other autophagy triggers are overused, they can actually cause illness rather than preventing or curing it. This being the case, it's important to progress to extreme fasts gradually, and never put yourself through more than three extreme fasts (exceeding twenty-four hours) per year without the advisement of a medical professional. Furthermore, it's best to practice intermittent fasting mindfully, with planning, purpose, and full comprehension of its potential effects on your body. Overachievers, beware! This is not a realm in which you should aim to be competitive or break records. Too much autophagic activity may be just as dangerous, if not more, than too little.

May cause undesired weight loss

Some demographics, including the elderly, women who are pregnant or nursing, cancer patients, and more, truly cannot afford to lose too much of their body fat. While fasting isn't the only way to bolster autophagy, it is the primary and most effective method, and all other methods also boost weight loss. For some people, it may not be worth the risk of undernourishment.

Risk of developing gallstones

Any lifestyle change that involves extreme or rapid weight loss and toxin elimination puts stress on the gallbladder. This is because the liver is releasing a higher than average amount of cholesterol into the gallbladder in the form of bile, which the gallbladder then stores, planning to reuse it for digestive purposes in the future. But if you are losing weight *and* regularly fasting, that bile ends up sitting in the gallbladder, unmoving and undisturbed, for longer than it's typically meant to. Under these circumstances, that bile can become highly saturated, dense, and eventually crystallize, forming painful gallstones. There may be steps you can take to counteract this risk, but anyone with a previous history of gallbladder issues should avoid fasting unless otherwise advised by their doctors.

Gender inequality

There is some concern within the health and wellness community that fasting—whether intermittent or extreme—may have differing effects on men and women, and some especially negative effects on female health. Autophagy induction alters hormonal activity, which can influence mood, appetite, sleep cycles, reproductive function, and energy levels. This hormonal shift is often described in a positive light by fasting and autophagy enthusiasts, but because the standards vary between genders, women unfortunately run a higher risk of overdoing it when they aim to activate the autophagic process, sending themselves into a period of hormonal imbalance. Autophagy promotes heightened levels of testosterone in particular, which may not be ideal for some women.

Cancer treatment may backfire

While it is admittedly exciting to imagine the potential of controlled autophagy to serve as the secret ingredient in a cancer cure, it's important to recognize the risks of inducing autophagy while hosting malignant cancer cells. These cancerous cells may take advantage of the process of autophagy just like healthy cells would, making themselves stronger and more efficient, causing tumors to grow even larger and more aggressive, and even allowing them to become resistant to traditional cancer treatments, such as chemotherapy.

Risk factors

While the potential benefits may sound tempting, certain people are advised to avoid fasting and extreme exercise to induce autophagy (unless advised otherwise by a medical professional), such as...

- Women who are pregnant

- Women who are currently breastfeeding

- Individuals diagnosed with diabetes or hypoglycemia

- Anyone who is struggling, or has formerly struggled, with an eating disorder, or severe body image distortion, such as body dysmorphic disorder

- Endurance athletes (unless under advisement)

- The very young

- The elderly

- Any individual who is already underweight

- Those with hormone conditions that provide an overabundance of testosterone

- Anyone dealing with mental health conditions that involve obsessive thought patterns or compulsive behaviors

- Anyone with health conditions that involve a low white blood cell count

Chapter 4: Fasting—how to begin, and what to expect

There are a number of factors that contribute to the improved function of autophagy, but if your objective is to push it from maintenance mode to a stress-response mode (which is more effective in combatting health threats, weight gain, and signs of aging) the most effective method is periodic nutrient starvation—also known as intermittent fasting. Extreme fasting, or prolonged fasting, is also effective, but it's highly recommended that you practice intermittent fasting first, in order to prepare your body and mind for such an intense experience.

When beginning a fasting regimen, planning is key. Otherwise, you are likely to incur unexpected hormone fluctuations, blood sugar spikes and energy crashes, mood swings, possibly even headaches and nausea. You'll want to ease into this if it's your first time fasting; don't schedule your first day of caloric restriction on your first day at a new job, or the same day on which you've agreed to help a friend move several large pieces of furniture into a five floor walk-up apartment. You won't want to attempt your first fast while suffering from a hangover, or while you're still recovering from a cold or flu. Fasting can also temporarily raise your heart rate, making you irritable and short-tempered; this being the case, you may want to avoid fasting through celebratory events like weddings or birthday parties, at least if you care about making a good impression on the people around you. You may also want to avoid fasting while enduring a period of intense emotional upheaval or grief.

Instead, you'll want your first fast to be well planned. Know what time you plan to stop eating, and what time you plan to break the fast; know what you plan to eat when the fast is over, so you won't binge on sugar, or make other unhealthy choices that undo all the potential benefits of autophagy immediately after inducing it.

You'll also want to prepare yourself mentally for the challenge. Especially if you've lived on a high-carb or high-sugar diet in the past, it will take some time for your body to adjust to a lifestyle that promotes enhanced autophagy, and the transition period can be vexatious. Your cells will go through a form of withdrawal, and will initially be sluggish to catch wise to the fact that there is less sugar in the bloodstream than they are accustomed to, slow to realize that they'll have to find alternative sources of energy. If this phase is particularly difficult or uncomfortable for you, rest assured— the symptoms of this withdrawal may be quite severe at first, but they will drastically improve once your body starts to get used to the new routine, usually after just a few days. Many people refer to this withdrawal as the "induction flu," and report that symptoms are worst on the 2nd, 3rd, and 4th days of autophagy activation. If you find that you're still suffering from low energy levels, headaches, nausea, mood swings or brain fog after a full week of intermittent fasting, it may be best to consult your physician before continuing with any type of fasting regimen to ensure there is no threat of health complications.

During the "induction flu," you may also experience some bizarre, uncomfortable, or painful physical sensations. For example: when autophagy works to burn excess fat in the body, it converts that fat into water, which is often flushed from the body in the form of perspiration or urine. When you begin fasting, you may find yourself sweating a great deal more than usual, as though jittery and anxious, or needing to use the bathroom every hour, even if you haven't consumed more water than you typically do. Headaches and nausea during fasting are usually either a symptom of stimulant withdrawal, or a sign that the body is dehydrated. To combat this, make sure you're drinking enough water to replenish your body as it works to flush out toxins; you may also want to add sea salt to the water you drink, or instead nurse a cup of bone broth, to ensure water retention and an adequate supply of necessary vitamins and minerals.

When your insulin begins to level out and metabolic function improves, you'll begin to gain enough control over your appetite and insight into its purpose to eventually be able to recognize the difference between a nutrient craving, a hunger pang, and a lust for comfort food. When we eat three standard meals a day, beginning shortly after waking and finishing our last meal just before bed, usually with plenty of snacks and calorie-packed beverages to string us over between meals, most of us never have enough time away from food to learn the difference between these sensations. Once you begin fasting, though, you will quickly begin to understand the power of food chemistry and the human appetite, and the effects these things have on your state of consciousness.

To our bodies, food is more than just fuel—the way we eat, the nutrients we choose, and the timing of our consumption all influence the way we think, and ultimately, the ways in which we behave. When you begin fasting, and your cells and brain begin to fall out of their usual rhythm of energy consumption, they'll become convinced that there is a scarcity problem, assuming your lack of caloric intake is due to a lack of nutritional availability. They will quickly begin to prepare you to survive a famine, enhancing your sense of smell, sight, and hearing to prime you for a hunt; this being the case, you might begin to take note, for the first time, of the particular sound that bacon fat makes when it sizzles and pops in a hot pan, or how loudly your co-workers chew on their sandwiches at lunchtime. You may notice odors in your kitchen that you'd never been aware of before; that includes both good and bad smells, so you might find yourself sniffing out that one rotten blueberry that rolled under your couch last month, or the closed jar of sauce in your refrigerator that's just starting to turn rancid.

The sight or odor of particular types of food may become so overpoweringly tempting as to become distracting, possibly even triggering drastic emotional responses. You might find yourself filled with genuine anguish and despair as you drag yourself out of a coffee shop with nothing but green tea in your hand, narrowly escaping the alluring scent of cinnamon buns and breakfast sandwiches unscathed. Alternatively, you might find yourself bursting with pure, unadulterated joy when your scheduled fast is over and it's time to feast—the kind of joy that would usually come from a promotion or wedding or new baby, as though securing food for dinner is an accomplishment worthy of exuberant celebration.

It is no coincidence that taste and smell are so closely linked, or that our mouths begin to produce saliva whenever we see or smell a particularly enticing treat, whether its sweet or savory; our bodies are designed for hunting and gathering, built to recognize feasting opportunities and take advantage of them. But we no longer live in a world of caloric scarcity or survival stress, so in comparison to our nomadic ancestors, we can afford to be much more selective with our diets, less reactive and less opportunistic. This means we can use strategic fasting and other forms of autophagy activation to train our minds to dismiss certain impulses triggered by food temptation. After weathering the "induction flu," many people report that their desires for carbohydrates and sugar quickly become much less intense, as does their tolerance overly sweet and processed foods.

Candies, pastries, and cookies that once seemed palatable will suddenly taste as though they've been injected with twice the normal amount of sugar, and eating them might even give you an intense sugar rush or even a sudden wave of nausea.

Through fasting, you'll experience three different forms of food desire. The first, and often hardest to ignore, is lust for comfort; this is the feeling of wishing you could sink your teeth into a stack of pancakes smothered in syrup and whipped cream. It will take some time to learn that this feeling is not usually related to authentic hunger; more likely, it is correlated to sugar addiction (glucose is an addictive substance, just like caffeine or nicotine) and feelings of anxiety. There is a reason we call carbohydrate-dense and sugar-loaded dishes "comfort foods"—they often leave us in a food coma afterwards, too numbed and exhausted to deal with the sources of our stress. These are the foods we consume to escape boredom, dull emotional pain, justify procrastination, or create a sense of security in our lives. After regular fasting and activation of autophagy, you'll begin to recognize that these are not the foods that our bodies truly want—they primarily exist to fulfill our emotional desires.

The second form of food desire is a genuine hunger pang. The human body is designed to withstand regular periods of fasting, so many of us won't experience this sensation until the late stages of a short fast, usually more than eight hours after consuming our last meal. The timing will depend upon the frequency with which you usually eat, as you will have previously trained your body to expect feeding at fairly regular intervals. One difference you may note is that hunger pangs are a much more physical experience than lust for comfort food; you may feel it in the depths of your gut, rather than primarily in your salivating gums, nostrils, or preoccupied mind. You may also note that there doesn't need to be any source of temptation present to trigger these feelings. Even without smelling food or seeing it, hunger pangs will push your brain to think about food. What's more, they may promote very specific and organized thought patterns regarding how to secure your next meal, how you'll prepare it, and precisely what nutrients will be best suited to satiating your appetite.

This brings us to the last form of food desire: nutrient cravings. When we free our bodies from glucose addiction and manufacture the conditions of nutrient scarcity, our cells can do an amazing job of communicating their specific nutritional needs to the brain. This happens to an extreme degree when women become pregnant; a fetus is weak and vulnerable to toxins that most adults can consume without problem, so the body uses tools like morning sickness (or generalized nausea at any time of day or night), extreme food aversions, and unusual cravings to steer the mother away from potentially toxic foods, and towards the particular nutrients that are needed for healthy fetal development. When fasting, once you move past any symptoms of withdrawal, you may experience powerful urges to eat very specific food groups. Strangely, you might find yourself craving fruits, vegetables, and proteins more than the comfort foods you're usually drawn to. Aim to honor these cravings when your fasting period comes to an end, as they may very well be indications that your body requires certain vitamins and nutrients to further its own healing process.

Our eating habits can shape our perceptions of the world around us; by activating autophagy through fasting and other habits, we can take control of this influence and our relationship to food, rather than allowing ourselves to remain stuck on the rollercoaster of blood sugar spikes and opportunistic consumption. It may be initially unpleasant, but ultimately, well-planned fasting can be a first step in the direction of a lifetime of improved health.

Chapter 5: Autophagy for your lifestyle

Induced autophagy is fairly difficult to achieve even when it is your primary focus. As with any lifestyle or dietary change, it can become even more challenging to sustain these habits once things like your work schedule, family, errands, or emotional distress, start to get in the way.

Many people who are interested in the benefits of autophagy are turned off by the idea of extreme or intermittent fasting, especially when they have hectic schedules to manage. It's understandable; for most of the twentieth century, we (along with the people that raised and educated us) were led to believe that all our energy comes from caloric intake, plain and simple. In fact, most of us were taught that carbohydrate consumption was the easiest, quickest, and healthiest way to get an energy boost; that protein consumption would always lead to muscle growth; and that fat was something to avoid at all costs, because it would slow the body down while fattening it up. We've been taught that more sleep is always better for us, and that exercise should be performed as frequently as possible. And furthermore, we've been taught that stress is the number one enemy of beauty, physical wellness, mental health, and longevity.

In truth, though, most of this is misinformation. Through the study of autophagy, we learn that when it comes to metabolic and cellular health, the devil truly is in the details. Timing matters. Moderation is key. Carbohydrate consumption can make us sleepy, while fasting can actually work to make us more alert. Macronutrient specificity can have a greater impact on the body than simply measuring the number of calories consumed versus number of calories burned through exercise. Too much exercise can actually be damaging, as can an overabundance of sleep, or a total absence of stressors. And of course, while occasional extreme fasts, or regular intermittent fasts, can be immensely beneficial, too much fasting can be detrimental to one's health, and indeed quite dangerous.

The good news is that autophagy can be triggered by a number of lifestyle habits beyond extreme fasting, many of which can be easily incorporated into even the most fast-paced lifestyles and chaotic schedules. It isn't only accomplished by restriction and reduction. Restorative sleep can help to induce autophagy (though you'll want to read up on what factors set you up for restorative sleep, versus non-REM sleep, which we'll explain in further detail in chapter 7), as can certain types of food (some of which is actually delicious and easy to acquire) and some supplements. Even a healthy sex life can boost the efficiency of autophagic activity in your body!

No matter what challenges your lifestyle poses, you can find a way to tap into the health benefits of increased autophagy without disrupting your schedule or abandoning other values. The important thing is to do it with purpose. Planning ahead will help you to maintain a balance, avoid over-fasting or over-exercising, and monitor your body's responses to specific stimuli. Every human body is different, so it may be wise to start slow, and adopt only one autophagy trigger into your lifestyle at a time, allowing you to pinpoint any practices that are incompatible with your body chemistry, your scheduling needs, or your personal goals.

Ten ways to induce and bolster autophagy

1 - Intermittent fasting

This is by far the most popular and oft-recommended method by which to activate autophagy. To use this tool effectively, you'll want to cut all sugars, carbohydrates, and proteins for 12 or more hours out of the day. Many people suggest aiming for 16-18 hours to hit the sweet spot for prime autophagic response, but you can do longer or shorter fasts and still see positive results.

If a 14 hour fast, for instance, sounds daunting, remember that you'll ideally be spending 6-8 of those hours sleeping, which leaves you with only 6-8 waking hours to pass without eating. Typically, people schedule their fasting hours in the morning so that they can feast in the evenings and promote restful sleep. This may also be done because it is often easier to get through a day of fasting when you know there is a feast to look forward to, a light at the end of the tunnel. For a 14 hour fast through the morning, you might eat dinner around 8pm or 9pm, and then stop consuming calories after 10 o'clock at night; sleep till 5 or 6 o'clock in the morning; skip breakfast (opting instead for a coffee laced with MCT oil or butter, or maybe a cup of autophagy promoting tea); and then finally break your fast with lunch at noon.

It may take some trial and error to find a routine that works well and is manageable for your lifestyle, but over time, you'll want to work up to a schedule of three or four consecutive fasting days, followed by several days of eating on a traditional, three-meals-per-day schedule.

2 - Protein cycling

You can use this tool in concert with intermittent fasting, combining both strategies to prime your body for major autophagic progress, but you can also use protein cycling in a traditionally scheduled meal plan to reap similar health benefits. By periodically limiting your protein intake to 25 grams or less over a twenty-four hour period, you'll force your cells to recycle or dispose of the protein that's already present in your body, encouraging the disposal of misfolded proteins that can build up and cause disease.

Imagine an irresponsible adult who's fallen into the habit of buying new socks and underwear every day because they can't be bothered to wash their own dirty laundry. Protein cycling is the equivalent of taking away that person's wallet, forcing them to make use of their own resources and develop some responsible habits before they purchase anything new.

Be advised, though—protein cycling should not be done every day or with too much frequency, as this can contribute to muscular degradation and actually speed up the aging process. Most people are able to incorporate protein cycling into an intermittent fast for three days out of a week without encountering any health risks, but if you are an endurance athlete, or someone who works in a physically demanding job position, you may want to cut back to just one or two days per week, ideally scheduling low-protein days on rest days, and consuming normal amounts of protein on days of heightened physical exertion.

3 - Extreme or prolonged fasting

As an alternative to intermittent fasting on a regular basis, you might choose to embark on two or three prolonged fasts annually. An extreme fast is one that exceeds 24 hours with no caloric intake that can trigger insulin response. Some may go on to fast for 36 hours, 48 hours, or even a full three days. Fasting beyond 72 hours without medical supervision is potentially dangerous, and not recommended for anyone in poor health or anyone without plenty of fasting experience under their belt. Extreme fasts exceeding 24 hours should not be undertaken more than three times annually without the approval of your doctor.

4 - Embracing the Ketogenic diet and lifestyle

For those who find fasting difficult to practice with any frequency, the Ketogenic diet may be the best dietary choice to promote autophagy, particularly for those who wish to combat and prevent neurodegenerative disease. This diet focuses on maintaining a strict balance of macronutrients in the diet at all times, regardless of how many calories are ultimately consumed, favoring fat as the largest source of caloric energy, with a moderate amount of protein and a very small amount of carbohydrates. Note that this diet measures net carbohydrates, meaning any carbohydrate that is offset by its own fiber content doesn't count towards the day's limit. It is not a no-carb diet, but rather a very, very low-carb lifestyle. When you consume lower amounts of carbohydrates, your body is forced to burn fat as an energy source, which puts the body into a state known as "ketosis." The ketogenic diet, or keto, as it's often called, is a very popular dietary tool to combat insulin resistance and prediabetes, as well as hormonal imbalances, neurodegenerative disorders like Alzheimer's, and even epilepsy in children. It is also an extremely popular diet for weight loss.

The ketogenic diet has a great deal in common with the paleo diet, with the major discrepancies lying in views on dairy consumption and methods of food preparation. While many people find it easier to stick to the ketogenic diet in the long term, as compared to any diet that suggests calorie reduction, getting started can be just as physically challenging as an initial fasting experience. To adjust to a lowered carbohydrate intake, the body goes through a period of withdrawal, known as the "ketogenic flu;" this involves all of the same symptoms you would encounter during an "induction flu," though they may be somewhat less severe when following a ketogenic diet.

5 - High intensity interval training

In adults, autophagy is best activated by pushing cells into stress-response mode. High intensity interval training, or HIIT, is an incredibly effective way to put cells under manufactured stress. HIIT has also been shown to boost function of the mitochondria and eliminate those which are no longer performing well, allowing every other part of the cell to function an enhanced level of efficiency.

With HIIT, a little goes a long way; only about 30 minutes of training is needed to achieve optimal results. By contrast, long distance endurance training does not seem to be able to provide similar benefits in terms of autophagic response. If weight loss, good health, and longevity are your primary motivations for exercise, then you may be better off embracing this less-is-more philosophy; skip the marathons, and instead reap these rewards from a just a couple hours of interval training per week. HIIT is usually recommended for 30 minutes, on 3 or 4 days out of every week; you might choose to use it every other day, making sure you leave time on alternate days for some resistance training and at least one twenty-four hour period of rest and recovery.

6 - Resistance training

As with most things in life, autophagy induced by exercise is best when used in moderation. Too much exercise, or too much autophagy, can actually lead to muscular atrophy, just as easily as too little. Resistance training is one way to ensure you're finding that ideal middle ground, prompting your body to source fuel from excess fat and damaged genetic material, rather than from the lean muscle that you want to hold onto. Autophagy is catabolic, so combined with only aerobic exercise and no strength training, it can be thrown into overdrive and become counter-productive to any goal besides weight loss—and since maintenance of a healthy weight is aided by lean muscle tissue, muscular degeneration and atrophy can also be counterproductive to achieving your weight loss goals.

There is also evidence to suggest that resistance training, unlike aerobic exercise, activates metabolic processes that signal autophagy activation and suppress mTOR.

7 - Restorative sleep

This recommendation should not be mistaken for a simple lecture about getting more shuteye. Some readers will indeed want to get more sleep to improve their overall health and stress levels, but too much sleep can actually work to interrupt autophagy. The goal is to find your own sweet spot—usually somewhere between six and eight hours per night—and aim to keep it fairly regular so that you can align your sleep schedule with your body's natural circadian rhythms.

To get restorative sleep, or deep REM sleep, you'll need to ensure your slumber is uninterrupted. That means no falling asleep in front of the television; those loud noises and bright lights are impacting your sleep quality, whether you're conscious of it or not. It also means conditions like sleep apnea, regular nightmares, or even excessive urges to eliminate waste in the middle of the night, should all be addressed. It may seem harmless to wake up once every night at two or three in the morning for a quick trip to the bathroom, but in reality, this interruption means there's a chance your deepest, most restorative sleep hours are being interrupted by bodily discomfort, and that is not ideal. If you wake up naturally in the middle of the night, there's nothing wrong with that at all—in fact, this may be a signal that your brain has completed a deep REM cycle, as it is quite normal to wake when shifting between phases of the sleep cycle. But if you are awoken in the night regularly and frequently, disturbed by ailments like nocturia, sleep apnea, or restless leg syndrome, it is very likely that you're getting too much light sleep and nowhere near enough restorative rest.

To ensure the best sleep quality, treat your bedroom like a cave or sanctuary; at bedtime, block out all sources of light and sound. During the evening, cut caffeine and try not to drink too many fluids right before bed. Smoking, alcohol abuse, and other habits that contribute to sleep apnea should be curtailed if possible. Dim technology screens in the early evening, and keep your eyes away from all bright screens for at least an hour before you retire. If all else fails, speaking to a cognitive behavioral therapist or sleep therapist can help you to combat insomnia and restructure your sleeping habits.

8 – Micronutrient management

If you've been living in a low-fat, high-protein, carbohydrate-craving mindset for a while, it may be time to think about redesigning the food pyramid in your head. The goal is to start thinking about these nutrient groups differently; you'll want to embrace the notion that fat is actually quite good for you when balanced correctly with other macronutrients, and that carbohydrates, while not necessarily bad for you, are not an ideal regular source of energy. Fat in food doesn't necessarily turn into fat inside the body, and it can be much more effective than carbohydrates at providing feelings of satiety and deep nourishment without causing insulin spikes or metabolic dysfunction. Following a ketogenic diet will prompt you to spend a great deal more time than you previously would have in examining food labels, becoming intimately familiar with the protein, fiber, sugar, carbohydrate, and fat contents in your favorite snacks; this can be a shock, initially, as you begin to realize that some vegetables, fruits, and "health" foods contain loads of sugar and carbohydrates, while some "junk" foods are actually a lot less harmful (fried pork rinds, for example, are a perfectly acceptable ketogenic snack, even if they are a cheap, gas station staple).

If you prefer not to follow the ketogenic diet strictly, you can still use macronutrient management strategically to promote autophagic activity by prioritizing fat consumption early in the day, and eating carbohydrates later in the afternoon or evening. This will help to train your body to look at fat as a long-lasting, sustainable energy source. Eating carbohydrates at night only can help to promote restful sleep, as well as preventing extreme hunger pangs upon waking the next morning.

Finally, if you find the idea of fasting or following any specific diet unrealistic or unmanageable, and can make only one lifestyle adjustment to promote autophagy, consider cutting sugar from your diet. When you start paying more attention to food labels, you will be shocked to see how much sugar is added to just about anything that is mass produced, including savory foods. Sugar is addictive, so one of the quickest and easiest ways to reduce appetite and insulin levels is to remove it from your diet. By reducing your sugar intake, you can improve your metabolic health drastically (and quickly), gaining more control over your energy levels and sleep cycle.

9 - Cellular stress

Alternating exposure to extreme hot and extreme cold can create exactly the type of cellular stress that boosts autophagy. You might accomplish this by switching back and forth between hot and cold water in the shower, or by jumping out of a hot tub into the snow. Some people like to spend time in saunas or steam rooms to manufacture cellular stress. As with all activities that induce autophagy, this should be practiced in moderation, and physical signs like nausea, dizziness, muscle cramps or severe headaches should be interpreted as a warning to pump on the breaks.

Another way to create stress at the cellular level is through hypoxia, which is a condition in which certain tissues within the body are deprived of adequate oxygen. Of course, it is extremely dangerous for any individual to deprive their own lungs of oxygen in hopes of achieving autophagy, but medical professionals may discuss targeted hypoxia in reference to new and experimental treatments to combat tumor growth and cancer development. Perhaps the only safe way for individuals to use hypoxia to their own advantage without incurring great risk to their own survival is to seize opportunities to exercise at high altitudes whenever possible. The lowered level of atmospheric oxygen at high altitudes will put additional strain on cells during physical exertion, but shouldn't pose any threat to your health so long as you stay below what mountaineers call "the death zone," starting at eight thousand meters above sea level, past which point the human body cannot acclimatize.

Any activity that is shown to stimulate the lymphatic system can help to promote cellular stress, and therefore trigger autophagy in turn. Even something as simple as eating spicy foods can help to accomplish this goal.

10 - Supplements, food ingredients, herbs and spices

There are plenty of ingredients and supplements that you can easily incorporate into your diet to boost autophagy. These include: caffeine, cinnamon, turmeric, ginger, green tea, apple cider vinegar, citrus, polyphenol supplements, resveratrol, Reishi mushroom extract, and nicotinamide.

Some autophagy enthusiasts make a point of drinking autophagy-promoting tea, or coffee boosted with butter and MCT oil, throughout the day, even during fasting periods, to stave off hunger and keep autophagic signaling active.

To make an autophagy promoting cup of joe, you'll want to skip any added milk or sugar. Start with a coffee bean you believe in—ideally, something organically grown and free of additives or toxins—and use healthy fats like grass-fed butter, organic coconut oil, MCT oil (MCT stands for "medium chain triglycerides") or a small amount of heavy whipping cream to enhance texture and flavor. Take care not to use more than 100 calories' worth of these added fats, otherwise you may risk negating the potential to trigger an autophagic response. Some people like to whip these liquids together with an electric mixer or handheld whisk to create a frothy, creamy layer of whipped fat at the top of the cup, like the dollop of foam in a traditional cappuccino. You could also add a dash of cinnamon to make your coffee even more effective at triggering an autophagic response—and quite a bit tastier, too. Cinnamon is effective at stabilizing insulin levels, and soothing some of the digestive discomfort that comes with drinking coffee, so it's highly recommended as a finishing touch for this recipe.

Autophagy tea leaves a bit more room for experimentation with flavor. You can brew a batch including as many or as few of the following ingredients as you like, depending on your taste preferences. Start with hot water and organic tea leaves (whether they're sold in tea bags or in loose leaf form doesn't matter); some people prefer to use green tea, while others prefer a citrus bergamot tea, like earl grey. Both types contain active polyphenols; if the flavors are compatible, you might even use both in the same pot! Be sure to let these tea leaves steep in the hot water for at least three minutes before removing them. You can feel free to let the tea leaves remain in the pot all day, too, extracting as many polyphenols as possible; over-steeping may result in a more intense or bitter flavor, but it also serves to make the tea even more effective at the work of promoting autophagy. You might also add cinnamon to this tea—ideally Ceylon cinnamon, which is the best quality cinnamon available—for its antioxidant properties. Organic coconut oil, turmeric, ginger, apple cider vinegar, and small amounts of unsweetened citrus juice are also fair game to add to this concoction, though you'll need to experiment to find the recipe proportions that are most palatable to you.

If autophagy tea doesn't sound appealing to you, there are other ways to get your fix of active polyphenols, which work to combat oxidative stress inside the body. You might find it easier to rely on daily supplements to source these, as well as curcumin (which is found in turmeric), resveratrol (found in red wine, the skin of most dark berries, peanuts and pistachios, soy, and dark chocolate), Reishi mushroom extract (only found in the medicinal mushrooms themselves), and nicotinamide (found in yeast, some meats and green vegetables).

Each of these supplements provides different benefits to your health, so ideally, you'd want to incorporate all of them into your diet to activate autophagy at every possible level. Be sure to keep your doctor informed about any supplements you take regularly, and take care not to overdose—in the world of vitamin and mineral supplements, too much of a good thing may prove to be worse for your body than inadequate amounts.

Bonus: two more strategies to trigger autophagic responses

All of the above listed strategies can be backed up with a fair amount of scientific evidence as to their effectiveness. Here are two more strategies for which there is supportive research—but that doesn't necessarily mean they won't work! Even if they aren't proven to promote autophagy in the end, they certainly can't do much harm.

Sexual activity

Luckily, not all of the stressors that help to promote autophagy are unpleasant! Studies suggest that regular sexual activity can help to stimulate autophagic processes. To reap the most autophagic benefits, aim to provide yourself with at least two hundred orgasms each year. Yes, that is a lot—one orgasm every 1.8 days—but there is no evidence to suggest that you'd need the participation of one or more partners to reach this goal. Autophagy can also be promoted through masturbation, so long as orgasm is achieved.

Facing stressors

This is by no means intended as an instruction to embrace chronic stress and anxiety, but rather a suggestion that you occasionally tackle and manage sources of potential stress, rather than avoiding them. This can be as simple as trying new things that are outside of your comfort zone once or twice a week; you might go to run an errand or out for a dinner date without a plan, forcing yourself to scramble and run around a bit; or alternatively, you might flirt with deadlines, prompting yourself to rush in order to meet them.

We often talk about how stressful modern life is, but perhaps we misuse the term in this context. Modern life is anxiety inducing, but in comparison to the forms of mortal stress our ancestors frequently weathered, most of us lead easy, breezy lives. We know where to find food and water; we don't worry every day about being attacked by hungry mammalian predators, or about having to find shelter in the event of a storm. You might think of these little controlled stress experiments as mental exercises; just as in physical exercise, you'll have to push yourself through a small amount of pain periodically to gain greater skill in the long-term. Eventually, enhanced autophagy will help you to naturally handle stress better, on both cognitive and physiological levels.

Lifestyle factors that inhibit autophagy

Processed foods

Preservatives and additives are not naturally occurring in our diets, so there's no reason why we should expect our bodies to be able to handle their digestion gracefully. Many of them include added sugars and artificially reduced fat content; this prompts insulin levels to rise to dangerous levels while leaving us less satisfied, leading us to quickly grow hungry for more caloric intake, even after we've just eaten.

Environmental toxins

From second hand smoke to pesticides to chemical pollutants, toxins in the environment cause an excess of oxidative stress within our bodies. Autophagy works to repair damage caused by free radicals, but too much exposure to these elements can overwhelm the system and ultimately render the process of autophagy ineffective.

Sedentary lifestyle

When we fail to practice regular exercise, we confuse our bodies. Food is meant to fuel us; if we eat consistently without burning the fuel, our cells become uncertain of what they're meant to do with all the excess energy in the body. Furthermore, by remaining inactive, we convince our brains, and even our individual cells, that there are no external threats to our survival; this then offers our autophagic pathways license to begin resting on their laurels and behaving as though they are part of a body that is much older than it actually is.

Fasting for any schedule

Some people may find it daunting to dive into a fasting regime, particularly those of us who aren't morning people, because the notion of skipping breakfast and coffee makes the idea of getting up almost unbearable. If your goal is to induce autophagy, though, you might be surprised to learn that this doesn't require you to fast on zero calories. In all the fasting schedules detailed below, we'll define fasting as a period during which you are not consuming any substantial amount of sugar, carbohydrates, or protein. Fat isn't necessarily off limits; nor is caffeine, or most herbs and spices.

Many people find it easier—and sometimes even pleasant—to adhere to a regular fasting schedule when they consume a small portion of fat in the morning, or sip on beverages throughout the day that contain some calories, but do not promote any kind of insulin response in the body or inhibit activation of autophagy. These beverages may include coffee, tea, sparkling water, apple cider vinegar, fatty oils (such as coconut oil or melted butter) or small amounts of citrus juice with no added sugar. Bone broth is also a popular choice for regular fasters, offering a savory, satisfying flavor to stave off hunger pangs without triggering an insulin response. It boasts a number of beneficial vitamins and minerals, and unlike coffee or tea, which are often diuretics, bone broth will help to keep you well hydrated due to its sodium content.

Then again, there are plenty of fasting enthusiasts who recommend working your way up gradually to a prolonged 72 hour fast, during which time you would consume nothing but water. Extreme as this may sound, it can help to truly break the body of many of its negative metabolic habits, shake addictions, promote mental clarity, purge toxins, and heal minor internal injuries. Some even claim that it can be a transformative and empowering emotional tool for reclaiming control of the body, freeing it from slavery to cravings and external stimulants.

That being said, expect extreme fasting to be both mentally and physically challenging, especially at first. You'll want to progress by small increments to prolonged fasting if you've never practiced it before; start with a series of shorter fasts, and work your way up to a 72 hour fast *only if* your body and mind respond positively to the experience.

Regular 12 hour fast

There is a high likelihood that you have already practiced a twelve hour fast a few times in your life without ever intending to. The breakfast meal earned its name for a reason; most of us don't consume any calories between bedtime and our first morning meal, and even when we are sleeping, our bodies can be triggered by nutritional deficiency to activate the autophagic process. A twelve hour fast is easily accomplished, either by cutting out post-dinner snacking, or by having breakfast after an hour or two of activity in the mornings. You could eat dinner at 7pm, finish all caloric consumption by 8 o'clock, then put yourself to bed by 10; sleep for seven or eight hours, get up by 6 o'clock, sustain yourself on coffee or tea for a couple of hours, and dig into your breakfast meal by 8am.

This moderate fasting period may not put your autophagic responses into extreme stress-response mode, but it will certainly be more beneficial than eating late at night, again first thing in the morning, and then snacking all day long. It's also a great way to adopt some discipline to your eating habits if your lifestyle involves a lot of stress, travel, or unpredictability, since it never requires you to count calories, eliminate common food groups, adhere to specific recipes, or search desperately for rare ingredients.

14-18 hour fast

Some wellness experts assert that this range is the sweet spot for women who want to induce autophagy, while it may lie beyond the 18 hour mark for men. This schedule can be designed quite similarly to the 12 hour fast, but with the breakfast meal skipped in its entirety; instead, a larger lunch meal would be the feast to break your fast. Some might prefer, instead, to eat an earlier dinner between 5 and 6 o'clock in the evening, waiting to eat until breakfast the next day at 8am (for a 14 hour fast), or until lunch at noon (for an 18 hour fast). This schedule may be particularly beneficial to those who wish to repair poor sleeping patterns, as digesting large quantities of food right before bed can lead some people to have disturbing dreams, restlessness, and indigestion, all of which may interfere with restorative rest and therefore inhibit autophagy.

Alternatively, you may still find time to consume three meals between fasting periods, but since they'll all be eaten so close together—all within a 6-10 hour window—your natural appetite signals will discourage you from overindulging during that timeframe (so long as you avoid sugars and processed carbohydrates, which can distort and even hijack your body's craving signals).

If you need an extra boost of encouragement to move beyond the 15 hour mark of fasting, it might help to know that consuming all your calories within an 8-9 hour window will have a significant beneficial impact on your cardiovascular health.

18-22 hour fast

This fast will usually involve skipping two meals in a twenty four hour period; or, if your appetite allows, you might consume two smaller-than-average meals during your 2-6 hours of caloric intake. For an intermittent fast of this length, adequate rest is imperative; therefore, you may want to choose the specific meals you eat, or feeding hours, based on your personal experience with digestion and its impact on your sleep patterns.

Time restricted eating

In practical terms, there isn't much difference between intermittent fasting and time restricted eating; the primary difference lies in the way that we conceptualize the concept of limiting caloric intake through timing, rather than focusing on quantity. Some people find it easier, and less mentally daunting, to think in terms of a restricted eating window, focusing on when they should eat, rather than focusing on how much time should be spent suppressing their cravings.

This strategy would allow you to adjust your eating schedule to adapt to external circumstances; for example, an individual aiming to consume all of their calories within a four hour window would be at liberty to begin that window at any time of day that suits their needs. Adjusting this timing may mean that fasting periods before and after are slightly shortened or lengthened, but if the time window for caloric consumption remains consistent, the fasting periods should balance out over time. There is no actual disparity between practicing daily sixteen hour fasts, and consuming all of your daily calories within an eight hour window of time; the only real difference is the way these terms and concepts impact your state of mind.

Many people find this idea much more approachable than scheduled fasting. An easy way to start is to first eliminate all snacking after dinner (that includes dessert, unfortunately) and eat nothing until breakfast the next morning; this should ideally set you up for a 10-12 hour fast, most of which will pass while you are sleeping. You can then gradually work to either move dinner to an earlier time, or to set breakfast back later in the day—you might even choose to skip breakfast entirely. During a restricted eating window, you should feel free to eat your fill, so long as you're avoiding processed junk foods, refined carbohydrates, and high sugar content.

24 hour fast

Referring to this as a 24 hour fast may serve to make the act seem more intimidating than it really is, which is why some fasting enthusiasts call it the "OMAD" fast instead. OMAD stands for "one meal a day," which is the easiest way to practice this fast. Start with breakfast, and then eat nothing until breakfast on the following morning; if you find it easier, you might instead go from lunch to lunch, or dinner to dinner.

Even after regular intermittent fasting, going a full day without food can be challenging. Try to remember that hunger is often a conditioned response, and its uncomfortable or distracting symptoms tend to come in waves that last no longer than five or ten minutes at a time. If you can persevere through those temporary hunger pangs by sipping on autophagy tea or bone broth, or even just taking a walk around the block to distract yourself, you'll most often find you are returned to a state of mental clarity and calm soon enough.

36 hour fast

A 36 hour fast will involve two sleep cycles without caloric intake. You might start in the evening after dinner, and wait until breakfast two days later to resume eating. Some autophagy enthusiasts believe that the 36 hour mark is the point at which stress-response mode autophagy is kicked up another notch, beginning to provide health effects that last for weeks or even months after the fast is completed.

2-3 day fast

If you're new to the world of prolonged fasting, it's imperative that you plan ahead and prepare yourself for this experience. Fasts of this length, particularly when undertaken for the first time, can be uncomfortable and downright painful if you do not set yourself up for success beforehand. Any addictions you have will come to the surface during a fast, including dependence on sugar, carbohydrate energy, caffeine, and more. Some people also report that time seems to slow during prolonged fasting, which could be viewed as a beneficial side effect, or a torturous one, depending on your attitude.

It's also important to be aware that prolonged fasting can temporarily reduce your white blood cell count by a drastic degree. Anyone with health conditions that may be complicated by a lowered white blood cell count should not attempt a prolonged fast without medical advisement or supervision.

Don't make the mistake of embarking on a prolonged fast without weaning yourself off of your usual caloric intake schedule first. In the 3 or 4 days leading up to the fast, make a point of gradually reducing the size of your meals, and ensure that your plate is full of nutrient-rich foods. Avoid processed foods, empty calories, sugar and alcohol to make the transition into your fasting period easier and prevent blood sugar crashes.

Prepare your living space, too. If you live alone (or with cooperative housemates who support your fasting goals) aim to clear your kitchen and refrigerator of visible temptations, and any foods with particularly strong odors. Your sense of smell will be enhanced, and you may even be able to detect scents that are emanating from sealed containers. Past the twenty-four hour mark, these scents, or even the mere sight of food, may become extremely tempting and distracting, so it may be best to keep them out of sight and out of mind for the time-being.

If you'll be consuming beverages aside from water, stock up on the coffee, tea, bone broth, fatty oils, herbs, spices and supplements you need beforehand, so you can avoid trips to the grocery store during the fasting period. If you plan to consume water only, you'll also want to stock up on high quality sea salt—not regular table salt. You'll add a pinch of salt to the water you drink in order to replenish your electrolytes and stay well-hydrated. The salt will also help to prevent nausea and dizziness during a prolonged fast.

During a prolonged fast, your body will be working hard to heal internal injuries, and expel toxins. This means that you might feel somewhat irritable, impatient, moody or jumpy during the fast, especially if it is your first time. This also means you should be prepared to feel, and smell, a little less clean and rosy than your usually self. Expect odorous perspiration, frequent urination, foul smelling breath and unusual bowel movements (unusual in the sense that they may come more frequently than you're accustomed to, and you may be expelling things that you didn't consume at any point in the recent past—don't be surprised to find strange colors, shapes, or textures in the toilet bowl).

When it's time to end your fast, resist the temptation to dive head first into an enormous meal of comfort food. Your body won't be ready to digest anything too complex at this point. Start small—ideally very small, with a cup of hot water and lemon juice to wake up your digestive organs and metabolism. Then, perhaps a handful of nuts, or small cup of yogurt. After this, wait for about an hour before attempting to eat again, giving your digestive system time to warm itself up and prepare for a larger meal. Make sure your first few full meals are small and low-glycemic, otherwise you may risk signaling your body to go into fat storage mode and sending your blood sugar levels into a tailspin. Once your gut is back in the swing of regular digestion, you can dig into a veritable feast, and congratulate yourself on a fast well done.

Chapter 6: Autophagy and weight loss

Our culture is obsessed with weight loss. It's fairly easy to see why; though many people are initially motivated to lose weight through a desire to improve their physical appearance, hoping to be seen as more attractive to others, over the course of a lifetime, the battle to keep off those extra pounds often transforms into a fight for survival. Doctors, nutritionists, trainers, and even people with no particular expertise in the health and wellness fields will encourage you to lose weight for the sake of your health, rather than in the name of vanity. No matter what relationship you have to your own body image, or how confident and comfortable you feel within your skin, the fact remains that carrying unnecessary excess weight places a great deal of stress on all the systems and organs in your body.

Obesity is a modern health epidemic that is linked to all sorts of unpleasant, painful, and potentially fatal chronic diseases. The National Institutes of Health posit that obesity is now the second leading cause of preventable deaths in the United States of America, coming in right behind tobacco use. It is a leading factor in metabolic dysfunctions (insulin resistance, hypoglycemia, diabetes), hypertension, liver and heart diseases, reproductive challenges, and even some mental health disorders. It is also believed to contribute to heightened cancer risks. In light of these facts, it's easy to see why the weight loss industry as a whole (including companies selling diet and meal plans, fitness regimes, miracle supplements and appetite suppressant pills, and more) is worth over seventy billion dollars in the United States alone, as of the year 2019.

And yet, even with all of that focus, attention, research, effort, and money being thrown at the problem, obesity rates in the United States only continue to rise. Data shows the epidemic is rapidly worsening, and the challenge of national obesity has recently been declared a public health crisis of graver consequence than the opioid epidemic. Currently, more than seventy percent of all adults in the United States are overweight or obese, and this percentage rate is expected to rise further in the next decade.

More than 45 million people in the United States embark on new diet and exercise regimes each year, many of them spending money on health plans that they frankly cannot afford to spare. Clearly, the desire to drop extra pounds and improve health outlooks is present; evidently, we are highly motivated to strive for significant change. So why is it the case, then, that approximately 97 percent of people who lose a significant amount of weight through caloric reduction and increased physical activity end up gaining it all back (and then some) within three years?

I'll repeat that to make sure it sinks in. In the United States, we are throwing more than seventy billion dollars annually at the obesity epidemic, and seeing less than a three percent success rate as a result. It seems fairly clear, then, that our traditional views on weight loss strategies (or, perhaps more importantly, strategies to keep the weight off once it's been shed) are not working. It also seems evident that weight loss shouldn't be our primary goal, as we have found many effective strategies for drastic weight reduction; instead, we should perhaps be focused on strategies to prevent morbid levels of weight gain in the first place, as well as strategies for maintaining healthy bodyweight once weight loss goals are achieved.

This is where autophagy can offer us hope for the future.

It may seem fairly obvious that fasting can aid in the weight loss process, since it involves severe caloric restriction. But it's important to note that induction of autophagy, which seems to lead to overall better weight loss results through less effort than most other diets, isn't just about reducing consumption. Instead, those who wish to use autophagy in efforts to slim down will want to focus on when they eat, and what macronutrients are consumed at what times, rather than how many calories are consumed in total. Timing and quality of nutrition both matter a great deal more than quantity.

Activating autophagy is a bit more complicated than simply eating less and exercising more, but when done thoughtfully and in healthy moderation, it should be an easier lifestyle change to sustain than extreme dieting or intense physical exertion. Autophagy can provide longer-lasting weight loss results because it trains the body and the mind to adjust positively to a healthier lifestyle, in contrast with diets that train the body to fear the sensation of satiety, ignore its own hunger signals, and focus obsessively on restriction, constraint, and denial of desires.

For those who have struggled with weight loss for years and practiced yo-yo dieting, the notion of regular intermittent fasting may be tough to embrace. Yo-yo dieting can do a real number on the metabolism over time, and cause to some uncomfortable and frightening symptoms in the body, leading us to fear any other extreme deviations from the traditional western diet. You might worry that fasting could cause a major blood sugar crash, which might involve nausea or vomiting, fainting, weakness and shakiness, muscle cramping, stomach pains, and more. You might also worry that it will lead you to binge to an unhealthy degree after your fasting period is over. Finally, you might just worry that the sensation of hunger experienced during a fast will be unbearable.

Surprisingly, though, many people who turn to autophagy activation for weight loss end up reporting that once they get past the initial hurdle of glucose withdrawal, they actually feel less hungry the more often they fast. This might sound counterintuitive, but it does make sense; through intermittent fasting, we can retrain most cells in our bodies to alter their caloric expectations. Unless we are living in a state of nutritional scarcity, most of us experience the symptoms of hunger as conditioned responses; we train our bodies to associate certain times of day or specific activities with the act of eating, triggering hunger signals when they are not biologically necessary for survival. Through autophagy, you can program your digestive organs and your cells to stop telling you that you're starving when you really aren't. Fairly quickly, intermittent fasting can start to feel comfortable and easily manageable; furthermore, as compared to other forms of dietary restriction, it can actually train your body to feel satiated with a much smaller number of calories, making weight loss a natural side effect of shifting appetite, rather than a constant struggle to ignore hunger signals. The concept of eating mindfully has been popular in weight-loss communities for decades; autophagy encourages not only mindfulness in eating, but also mindfulness in the experience of hunger, teaching us to better understand the messages our bodies send us, and removing factors that may serve to distort those messages, such as sugar addiction.

Furthermore, studies suggest that intermittent or prolonged fasting does encourage higher caloric consumption at the end of fasting periods—subjects in experiments would often eat twenty to twenty-five percent more calories at their fast breaking meal, compared to subjects who followed a traditional reduced calorie diet before being encouraged to eat their fill at the same meal period. So yes, fasting periods do increase our hunger levels, and prompt our bodies to feast afterwards—but these studies have also found that increased caloric intake after fasting typically does not offset the caloric deficit ramped up during the course of the fast. By fasting and feasting, subjects were able to report higher levels of satiety at their feasting meal, while still ultimately reducing their overall caloric intake over the course of the day (or in some cases, multiple days). This strategy becomes even more effective for those who are able to maintain a high-fat, low-carbohydrate and low-sugar diet in between fasting periods, as their metabolisms are better able to adapt to the unpredictable eating patterns.

When we promote autophagy through autophagy or ketosis, we also train our bodies to exhibit more metabolic flexibility. Yo-yo dieters are often fearful of fasting and feasting because they believe that extreme caloric restriction over extended periods can slow down the metabolism in a permanent way. But autophagy helps restore metabolic function and allows it to become adaptable and resilient without a predictable dietary schedule.

In the end, autophagy induction may be our best weapon to fight against the obesity epidemic because it involves sustainable lifestyle changes, encouraging rewards rather than prompting fear of punishment for falling off the wagon. Through autophagy, we can learn to make intuitive dietary choices that are positive for our unique body chemistries; we can reduce our reliance on scales to measure progress, and eliminate fear of muscle weight or water weight, slowed metabolisms, diet and exercise plateaus, lowered tolerance for restricted food groups and weight loss recidivism.

Chapter 7: Autophagy and the aging process

Age is defined by more than simply the number of times we've travelled around the sun. We all know that certain mile-markers of old age look and feel quite different from one individual to the next. There are plenty of fifty-year-old people out there with more wrinkles, sagging skin, grey hair, and liver spots than their elders; conversely, there are some seventy-year-olds who could literally run circles around people half their age, boasting radiant skin, clear vision and good hearing, internal balance and proprioception, well-functioning motor skills, and minds as sharp as tacks.

We all know that rates of cancer, chronic disease, and neurodegenerative disorder become more and more common in old age, and many of us are mindful to avoid lifestyle habits that might speed the development of such conditions; but what about those signs of aging that come inevitably, even if we remain in "good health" right up until the end of life? What do we really know, firmly, about the development of wrinkles and grey hairs? It seems fairly obvious that stress levels have something to do with these age signifiers, perhaps more than one's actual, biological age. We see this reality played out in the physical features of every United States president to take office and emerge, four or eight years later, looking as though they've fallen into a time machine and survived several decades of medieval era warfare before returning to us. At the same time, we also know that cellular stress promotes autophagy, which has been proven to suspend the aging process and all its physical signifiers in several animal species; therefore, stress can't be the only cause of such a transformation. Furthermore, we can observe that some people with drastically lower occupational stress levels also appear to age very quickly over short periods of time. For instance, many of us have known someone whose health and mental acuity began to decline rapidly after retirement, despite being perfectly functional beforehand.

So what, then, is the secret? Why do some of us age so much faster than others? And why does the aging process sometimes speed up, or slow down, so unpredictably?

It seems that autophagy may play a key role, not only in preventing diseases that speed aging and promote cellular death, but also in slowing the development of inevitable aging signifiers. A specific type of autophagy that works to keep all the mitochondria in the body functioning at their highest level of efficiency (a process known as mitophagy) seems to be particularly relevant to the aging process, as mitochondrial decline leads to lowered energy levels and overall cellular deterioration. But more than likely, autophagy works on multiple levels to combat aging, some of which we have not yet adequately studied or even discovered.

Wrinkles, Skin discoloration, and dryness

Your skin is made of a number of elements, but 75 to 80 percent of the organ is all collagen. Collagen is what makes your skin firm, smooth, and tight, but it is weakened by oxidative stress and free radical damage over time, which allows wrinkles to form. Autophagy works to negate the effects of oxidative stress, maintaining the skin's moisture levels and elasticity. It helps to prevent dehydration and discoloration by keeping your collagen levels stable, which allows the skin to function as a secure barrier against external stressors like harsh light, air pollutants, and other free radical sources, while keeping moisture sealed within.

Grey hair

There is some evidence to suggest that premature greying or thinning of the hair is primarily caused by genetic inheritance, but autophagic activity rates may also play a role here. We often associate premature greying with high levels of stress in our lifestyles, but it seems that nutrition and vitamin sufficiency may actually be the most influential factors, since high-stress is often correlated with impulsive and poor dietary choices. With an overabundance of caloric intake and a lack of adequate autophagy, senescent cells are allowed to remain dormant in the body, instead of being degraded and recycled or disposed of, and they can build up; these senescent cells release inflammatory cytokines and interrupts a number of biogenetic processes in the body, including the production of melanin, which is responsible for hair color.

Sleep

When we are infants, we can spend up to half of our time asleep in the REM state, which provides the most restorative and rejuvenating benefits; but as we age, we gradually lose the ability to make the most of our slumbering hours. The average adult getting eight hours of shuteye each night is likely in REM sleep for only two of those hours, on average, compared to the four hours of restorative sleep that a baby would get. This ratio can decrease even further as you progress into old age, especially if your slumbering hours are more frequently interrupted by factors like sleep apnea, acid reflux, or chronic pain, meaning that even when you get a full eight hours (or more) of sleep in old age, you may still be at risk for suffering the long-term health effects of chronic sleep deprivation. Without adequate restorative sleep, our immune systems grow weaker; many types of inflammation are allowed to thrive and spread throughout the body; weight gain and metabolic dysfunctions are encouraged; organ functions begin to fall into decline (including skin, which is also an organ—this may be why sleep deprivation appears to be correlated to development of wrinkles); and finally, memory and cognitive functions are weakened.

Any steps we can take to improve sleep quality and increase duration of restorative rest can work to promote autophagy, counteracting these undesirable effects. Beyond fasting, autophagy works best during deep sleep.

Motor Function

Autophagy appears to play a protective role in the brain, shielding the neurons responsible for directing motor activity from potentially damaging protein buildup and loss of synaptic plasticity.

Osteoarthritis

Studies have found that many patients suffering from osteoarthritis in old age are also dealing with suppressed expression of the genes that trigger autophagy in the body. By working to purposefully activate it, patients may be able to counteract this internal deficiency and soothe inflammation and pain associated with the disease, or even prevent its development before it can progress to a severe state.

Brain health

One of the most exciting and promising features of autophagy is its beneficial impact on the brain, primarily as a shield against neurodegenerative disorders that typically emerge in old age. We'll touch on this in more detail in the 9th chapter.

Longevity

One thing we still do not fully understand about autophagy is why the process naturally slows, or becomes less effective, as organisms age. We can introduce manufactured cellular stress to re-activate it, but scientists are still looking for answers as to why it needs to be tampered with at all. In 2009, a research team at Osaka University discovered Rubicon, a protein factor that appears to cause increased autophagic inhibition with age in animals, and they were able to show that by reducing Rubicon expression rates in model organisms (rodents, insects, and worms) they could promote autophagy, reducing symptoms of aging such as declining motor function and fibrosis. Amazingly, they were also able to prove that Rubicon suppression and autophagic promotion can prolong the aging process, allowing these animals to survive for much longer than they otherwise would have.

Rubicon can be suppressed through restricted caloric intake, leading to extended lifespans and fewer measurable signs of aging. But again, this finding only shows us a correlation, not necessarily proving causation, nor explaining why Rubicon suppression doesn't occur naturally in living organisms.

If our cells all come programmed with their own internal self-cleaning mechanism, and all the tools necessary to repair themselves and extend their own lifecycles, why aren't they able to continue doing so indefinitely, without prompting or intervention?

It's entirely possible that we'll never find a conclusive answer to this question. If we can, though, that answer may lead us to solve one of life's greatest inherent mysteries: the meaning and purpose of death.

Chapter 8: Autophagy and health disorders

The discovery of autophagy, as well as the genetic components that govern the process, has the potential to change the face of medical science as we know it. While there have not yet been any clinical trials performed on humans—most thus far have been performed on rodents, insects, or microscopic organisms—there is a great deal of evidence to suggest that autophagic activity works to combat inflammation, obesity, buildup of toxins and misfolded or poorly built proteins, and metabolic dysfunction, all of which are known to contribute to development of chronic disease.

When you've been ill in the past, perhaps you've heard the common, but ultimately misleading, recommendation: "Starve a fever," people probably told you, "but feed a cold." On this advice, you might have bundled yourself up at home and feasted on chicken noodle soup for days at a time, believing in its mythical healing powers.

In truth, though, humans are the only mammals that push themselves to eat anything at all during illness or recovery from severe injury. While we usually are only hindered by illnesses that include nausea or indigestion, most other animals recognize that anytime the body is in recovery, it needs to divert all available energy to the healing process. The digestive system is somewhat narcissistic, as a whole; it is self-serving, and will rarely miss an opportunity to make itself the center of attention. Whenever it is active, it draws energy away from other systems and processes in the body, no matter how necessary or urgent they may be. So other animals—who are apparently wiser than us in many respects, however small their brains might be—subject themselves to periods of fasting and rest automatically when they are sick or hurt, allowing their bodies to channel all of their energy into a streamlined healing process.

It stands to reason, then, that fasting can have extraordinary powers for natural healing. At this time, there are not enough conclusive studies or experiments in existence to tell us for certain whether or not autophagy induction through fasting can be used to cure any particular ailments, disorders, or diseases, but there is plenty of evidence to suggest a correlation between inhibited autophagy and illness, as well as correlation between activated autophagy and recovery, plus strengthened immunity and prevention of disease recurrence. Again, we cannot yet say that there is solid proof of autophagy's healing or preventative capabilities, because correlation does not necessarily imply causation. But in the face of cancers and modern health disorders for which we have not yet found cures, a great number of people have decided that, despite the lack of proof, autophagy induction is certainly worth a try.

Autophagy to combat toxins and infectious disease

Autophagy is a powerful tool for detoxification. As mentioned in previous chapters, it works to detect free radicals and other suboptimal organic matter in the body, and then sequesters it (protecting other cells from corruption), degrades it (rendering this suboptimal matter into less of a potential threat to other cells) and repurposes it (often converting it into energy that can be directed towards other healing processes).

When it comes to viral infection, autophagosomes are experts at recognizing the particles that have no rightful place in the body. They aid in degradation of these particles, and furthermore, they trigger immune responses throughout the rest of the body to ensure that the threat will be found, addressed, and dismantled in a timely manner. Unfortunately, some powerful viruses are able to trick the autophagic process into helping them to survive and grow alongside healthy cells, or even to treat the healthy cells as the truly threatening outliers.

Autophagy and cancer

When looking at potential cancer treatments and preventative health measures, autophagy may be used as a powerful secret weapon with enormous beneficial properties. But just like powerful weapon, autophagy can also become quite dangerous if allowed to fall into the wrong hands. Just as it can be hijacked by some viruses, autophagy can sometimes be taken advantage of by cancerous or mutated cells.

To discuss the potential benefits of autophagy as a cancer preventer, let's examine a study done on fasting, autophagy, and breast cancer recurrence rates. This is one of very few studies on autophagy to involve human subjects, so the results are both astonishing and immensely valuable. In 1995, researchers began collecting data samples from over 2400 women who had previously been diagnosed with breast cancer; none of these women had diabetes; they represented a wide demographic group, ranging from the age of 27 to 70 years old. These women were asked to undergo nightly fasting, and their health outcomes were recorded for a subsequent number of years (11 years on average, but this varied from subject to subject). The study concluded that fasting for 13 hours or more on a nightly basis had reduced the rate of cancer recurrence for these subjects by forty percent.

If that fact alone hasn't knocked your socks off yet, let me add that these subjects were only prompted to reduce the number of hours per day during which they ate. They weren't discouraged from eating sugars or carbohydrates; they weren't prohibited from eating processed junk foods; they weren't required to maintain any sort of exercise regimen; and they weren't instructed to reduce or limit overall caloric intake.

As impressive as these findings might be, we must remember that these results were only consistently found in subjects who did not have any malignant cancer cells at the start of the study. For patients actively fighting cancer, autophagy may be too risky, as it can actually strengthen cancer cells and lead them to develop resistance to chemotherapy and radiation treatments. In fact, blocking or suppressing autophagic responses has, in some cases, been shown to help weaken a tumor's resilience and ability to cope with stress, helping chemotherapy treatments to finally kill the cancer cells off, despite former resistance to treatments.

Future research and experimentation will hopefully serve to guide us to a definitive answer; in the meantime, despite the lack of a cure, our discoveries about autophagy have provided us with invaluable insight into the behavior and development of cancer and all forms of malignancy in the human body.

Chapter 9: Autophagy and the mind

There is a great deal of evidence to suggest that autophagy is one of our best preventative defenses against many neurodegenerative disorders, including Parkinson's, Alzheimer's, and Huntington's disease. While Autophagy does not usually occur within brain cells, which are thought to be immune to metabolic processes that impact the rest of the body, it does work to rid us of the buildup of damaged, noxious proteins around the neurons that often cause these diseases. Unlike with viral infections or cancerous cells, there is no risk that autophagy will instead promote further growth of these harmful proteins. Therefore, the potential benefits are quite promising.

Neuroplasticity is central to cognitive function; it references the brain's ability to adapt to changing external factors, learn new skills, retain memories, and even recover after a brain injury. It is typically weakened with age, whether neurodegenerative disorders are present or not. But autophagy promotes enhanced neuroplasticity, not only by removing proteins that interrupt neural connections, but also by stimulating growth of matter that can be transformed into brand new neural cells. Over time, this allows the brain to continue functioning like a young organ, despite its true age.

Autophagic triggering, particularly through fasting or maintenance of a low-carbohydrate, low-sugar diet, can help to prevent or delay the onset of dementia in old age. There is also plenty of evidence to suggest that autophagy expression is required in order for the brain to create and retain memories. Some people may be able to use autophagy triggers in order to recapture memories lost due to old age or even brain injury.

Patients are often able to achieve better results through a combination of dietary change, increased physical activity, and other forms of manufactured cellular stress, rather than through fasting or macronutrient management alone. This being the case, it may make more sense to adopt a lifestyle that promotes autophagic activity earlier in life, so that you may prevent the onset of neurodegenerative disease entirely, rather than waiting to combat cognitive dysfunction at a point in life where the body may not be primed to handle physical stressors.

Conclusion

Thank you for making it through to the end of Autophagy: 10 powerful secrets of healing and anti-aging. Let's hope it has been informative and able to provide you with all of the tools you need to achieve your goals, whatever they may be.

The next step is to experiment with induction of autophagy to discover which habits can fit comfortably in your lifestyle, as well as which seem to provide you with the most desirable health benefits. Again, I'll reiterate that it's important to consult your doctor or a trusted health professional before diving into any extreme fasting practice, intense exercise regimen, or drastic alteration of your sleep schedule. Autophagy is a relatively new discovery in the field of medical science, and the activities that trigger it may indeed be risky for people with certain health conditions.

That being said, moderate experimentation with activation of autophagy can be an excellent way to get to know your own body better, and at the end of the day, you will have to be the one to decide what's best for it. Doctors can be brilliant healers, but they are merely human, and thus fallible and susceptible to influence from pharmaceutical companies, ever-changing dietary trends, and their own internal prejudices. No doctor will ever be able to understand your body as thoroughly as you can yourself, once you learn how to listen to it, and monitor its reactions to different stimuli.

Finally, if you found this book helpful, a review is always appreciated!

www.ingramcontent.com/pod-product-compliance
Lightning Source LLC
Chambersburg PA
CBHW070039230426
43661CB00034B/1436/J